Haircare Secrets of Ayurveda: Remedies for Hair Loss and Regrowth

Introduction

Hair loss is a common concern that affects millions worldwide, often leading to frustration and a search for effective solutions. Amidst the plethora of modern treatments, Ayurveda offers an alternative approach deeply rooted in ancient wisdom and natural principles. In this book, we delve into the realm of Ayurveda, exploring its time-honored practices and remedies for addressing hair loss in the modern era. By blending ancient wisdom with contemporary concerns, we uncover the transformative potential of Ayurveda in healing hair loss and promoting long-term hair health. Join us on a journey to rediscover the ancient practices that offer hope and holistic healing for modern hair concerns.

Chapter 1

Introduction to Ayurvedic Hair Care: Understanding the Principles

In the vast landscape of holistic healing traditions, Ayurveda stands out as a comprehensive system that encompasses every aspect of human health, including hair care. This chapter serves as a foundational exploration into the principles of Ayurvedic hair care, providing readers with a nuanced understanding of its underlying philosophy and approach.

The Essence of Ayurveda:

Ayurveda, often referred to as the "science of life," traces its origins back thousands of years to the ancient civilization of India. At its core, Ayurveda embodies a holistic understanding of the human body, mind, and spirit, emphasizing the interconnectedness of all elements within the universe. Central to Ayurvedic philosophy is the concept of balance, wherein optimal health is achieved through harmonizing the three doshas: Vata, Pitta, and Kapha.

The Doshas and Hair Health:

In Ayurveda, the doshas serve as dynamic forces that govern various physiological functions, including hair growth and maintenance. Understanding the unique qualities and characteristics of each dosha is crucial for comprehending how imbalances can manifest as hair-related concerns. For instance, excess Vata may lead to dryness and brittle hair, while aggravated Pitta can result in inflammation of the scalp and premature graying. Similarly, imbalanced Kapha may manifest as excessive oiliness and stagnation, contributing to conditions like dandruff and hair loss.

Holistic Healing for Hair:

Unlike conventional approaches that often focus solely on external symptoms, Ayurvedic hair care adopts a holistic perspective that addresses the root cause of hair-related issues. By identifying and rectifying imbalances at their source, Ayurveda seeks to promote sustainable and long-lasting solutions for hair health. This holistic approach extends beyond the physical realm to encompass mental, emotional, and spiritual well-being, recognizing the profound interplay between these aspects and overall hair health.

Ancient Wisdom, Modern Relevance:

Despite its ancient origins, Ayurvedic principles remain remarkably relevant in today's world, offering timeless wisdom that transcends cultural and temporal boundaries. In an era marked by the proliferation of synthetic products and quick-fix solutions, Ayurveda advocates for a return to nature and the utilization of natural remedies derived from plants, minerals, and herbs. By embracing Ayurvedic hair care practices, individuals can embark on a journey of self-discovery and empowerment, reclaiming agency over their hair health in alignment with the rhythms of nature.

As we embark on this journey into the realm of Ayurvedic hair care, it is essential to approach with an open mind and a willingness to embrace holistic healing modalities. By understanding the foundational principles of Ayurveda and their application to hair health, readers will gain invaluable insights that can revolutionize their approach to hair care. In the chapters that follow, we will delve deeper into specific remedies, practices, and lifestyle recommendations, guiding readers on a path towards vibrant, lustrous hair rooted in the wisdom of Ayurveda.

Chapter 2

Understanding Hair Loss: Causes and Contributing Factors

Hair loss is a multifaceted concern that affects individuals of all ages and backgrounds, often eliciting feelings of frustration and self-consciousness. In this chapter, we delve into the intricate web of factors contributing to hair loss from an Ayurvedic perspective, shedding light on its underlying causes and manifestations.

The Ayurvedic View of Hair Loss:

In Ayurveda, hair loss is not viewed as an isolated issue but rather as a symptom of underlying imbalances within the body. According to Ayurvedic principles, the health of the hair is closely intertwined with the state of the doshas (Vata, Pitta, and Kapha), as well as the overall well-being of the individual. Imbalances in any of these doshas can disrupt the natural cycles of hair growth and lead to various hair-related concerns.

Identifying the Root Causes:

Ayurveda recognizes a multitude of factors that can contribute to hair loss, each stemming from imbalances in the doshas and aggravated by external influences. These include:

1. Stress and Anxiety: Chronic stress and emotional turmoil can disturb the delicate balance of the doshas, leading to hair loss and thinning.

2. Dietary Imbalances: Poor dietary choices and nutritional deficiencies can deprive the hair follicles of essential nutrients, impairing their function and vitality.

3. Toxic Buildup: Accumulation of toxins (ama) in the body due to poor digestion and lifestyle habits can obstruct the flow of nutrients to the scalp, hindering hair growth.

4. Hormonal Imbalances: Fluctuations in hormone levels, particularly elevated levels of Pitta, can exacerbate hair loss

and contribute to conditions like alopecia.

5. Genetic Predisposition: While Ayurveda acknowledges the influence of genetics on hair health, it emphasizes the role of lifestyle and environmental factors in modulating genetic expression.

Understanding Patterns of Hair Loss:

Ayurveda categorizes hair loss into distinct patterns based on the predominant doshic imbalance and the specific symptoms observed. These patterns include:

1. Vata-Type Hair Loss: Characterized by dryness, brittleness, and erratic hair growth, often exacerbated by stress and anxiety.

2. Pitta-Type Hair Loss: Manifests as inflammation of the scalp, excessive heat, and premature graying, aggravated by stress and dietary factors.

3. Kapha-Type Hair Loss: Marked by excessive oiliness, stagnation, and dandruff, exacerbated by poor circulation and dietary imbalances.

Holistic Approach to Hair Loss:

In addressing hair loss from an Ayurvedic perspective, it is essential to adopt a holistic approach that encompasses dietary modifications, lifestyle adjustments, stress management techniques, and targeted herbal therapies. By addressing imbalances at their root cause and supporting the body's natural healing processes, Ayurveda offers a comprehensive framework for promoting healthy hair growth and preventing further loss.

Chapter 3

Herbal Remedies for Hair Loss: Nature's Solutions

In the pursuit of healthy hair, nature offers a rich tapestry of botanical remedies that have been revered for centuries for their therapeutic properties. In this chapter, we delve into the realm of Ayurvedic herbal remedies, exploring the diverse array of plants, herbs, and botanical extracts that hold the key to combating hair loss and promoting regrowth.

The Power of Ayurvedic Herbs:

Ayurveda harnesses the potent healing properties of plants and herbs to address a myriad of health concerns, including hair loss. These herbal remedies are prized for their ability to nourish the scalp, strengthen the hair follicles, and balance the doshas, thereby facilitating optimal conditions for healthy hair growth. By incorporating these herbs into our hair care regimen, we can tap into nature's wisdom and unlock the transformative potential of herbal medicine.

Key Herbs for Hair Health:

1. Bhringraj (Eclipta alba): Known as the "king of herbs for hair," Bhringraj is revered in Ayurveda for its rejuvenating properties. It nourishes the scalp, promotes hair growth, and prevents premature graying, making it a cornerstone of Ayurvedic hair care.

2. Amla (Emblica officinalis): Rich in vitamin C and antioxidants, Amla strengthens the hair follicles, promotes shine, and stimulates growth. It also helps to balance Pitta dosha, making it particularly beneficial for individuals experiencing inflammation-related hair loss.

3. Brahmi (Bacopa monnieri): Brahmi is revered for its calming and cooling properties, making it ideal for soothing irritated scalp conditions and promoting relaxation. It strengthens hair roots, improves circulation, and enhances overall hair health.

4. Neem (Azadirachta indica): Neem is renowned for its antimicrobial and anti-inflammatory properties, making it effective in combating scalp infections and dandruff. It cleanses the scalp, removes excess oil, and promotes a healthy environment for hair growth.

5. Shikakai (Acacia concinna): Shikakai is a natural cleanser that gently removes dirt, oil, and buildup from the scalp without stripping its natural oils. It promotes lustrous hair, prevents dandruff, and strengthens the hair shaft.

Formulations and Applications:

Ayurvedic herbal remedies for hair loss can be prepared in various forms, including oils, powders, pastes, and decoctions. These formulations can be applied topically to the scalp, massaged into the hair, or consumed internally as part of a holistic approach to hair care. By tailoring the choice of herbs and formulations to individual needs and doshic imbalances, we can maximize their efficacy and achieve optimal results.

Recipes

1. Ayurvedic Herbal Hair Oil:

Ingredients:

- 1 cup coconut oil or sesame oil (base oil)

- 2 tablespoons dried Bhringraj leaves

- 2 tablespoons dried Amla powder

- 1 tablespoon dried Brahmi powder

- 1 tablespoon dried Neem leaves

- 1 tablespoon fenugreek seeds (optional)

Instructions:

1. In a clean, dry glass jar, combine the base oil (coconut or sesame oil) with the dried herbs and seeds.

2. Seal the jar tightly and place it in a sunny spot for 2-3 weeks to allow the herbs to infuse into the oil.

3. Shake the jar gently every day to ensure even distribution of the herbal extracts.

4. After 2-3 weeks, strain the oil using a fine mesh strainer or cheesecloth to remove the solid particles.

5. Transfer the infused oil into a clean, dark glass bottle for storage.

6. To use, warm a small amount of the herbal oil in your hands and massage it into your scalp and hair. Leave it on for at least 30 minutes or overnight for maximum benefits before shampooing as usual.

2. Ayurvedic Herbal Hair Mask:

Ingredients:

- 2 tablespoons Amla powder

- 2 tablespoons Brahmi powder

- 1 tablespoon Shikakai powder

- 1 tablespoon yogurt (optional, for additional conditioning)

Instructions:

1. In a small bowl, combine the Amla, Brahmi, and Shikakai powders.

2. If using yogurt, add it to the powdered mixture and mix well to form a smooth paste.

3. Apply the herbal hair mask to damp hair, starting from the roots and working your way to the ends.

4. Leave the mask on for 30-60 minutes to allow the herbs to penetrate the hair shaft and nourish the scalp.

5. Rinse the mask out thoroughly with lukewarm water, followed by a gentle shampoo and conditioner.

3. Ayurvedic Herbal Hair Rinse:

Ingredients:

- 2 cups water

- 2 tablespoons dried Hibiscus flowers

- 1 tablespoon dried Rosemary leaves

- 1 tablespoon Apple cider vinegar (optional)

Instructions:

1. Bring the water to a gentle boil in a small saucepan.

2. Add the dried Hibiscus flowers and Rosemary leaves to the boiling water.

3. Allow the herbs to steep in the water for 10-15 minutes, then remove the saucepan from the heat.

4. Let the herbal infusion cool to room temperature before straining out the herbs.

5. If desired, add the apple cider vinegar to the herbal infusion and mix well.

6. After shampooing and conditioning your hair, use the herbal rinse as a final rinse to restore pH balance, add shine, and promote scalp health.

4. Ayurvedic Herbal Hair Mask for Dry Hair:

Ingredients:

- 2 tablespoons coconut milk

- 1 tablespoon honey

- 1 tablespoon aloe vera gel

- 1 tablespoon avocado oil or olive oil

- 1 tablespoon Brahmi powder

- 1 tablespoon Hibiscus powder

Instructions:

1. In a small bowl, combine all the ingredients to form a smooth paste.

2. Apply the hair mask evenly to damp hair, focusing on the ends and any dry or damaged areas.

3. Leave the mask on for 30-60 minutes to deeply nourish and moisturize the hair.

4. Rinse the mask out thoroughly with lukewarm water, followed by a gentle shampoo and conditioner.

5. Ayurvedic Herbal Hair Rinse for Dandruff:

Ingredients:

- 2 cups water

- 2 tablespoons dried Neem leaves

- 1 tablespoon dried Tulsi (Holy Basil) leaves

- 1 tablespoon Apple cider vinegar

- 5 drops Tea tree essential oil (optional, for extra antifungal properties)

Instructions:

1. Bring the water to a gentle boil in a small saucepan.

2. Add the dried Neem leaves and Tulsi leaves to the boiling water.

3. Allow the herbs to steep in the water for 10-15 minutes, then remove the saucepan from the heat.

4. Let the herbal infusion cool to room temperature before straining out the herbs.

5. Add the apple cider vinegar and tea tree essential oil to the herbal infusion and mix well.

6. After shampooing your hair, use the herbal rinse as a final rinse to combat dandruff, soothe the scalp, and restore pH balance.

6. Ayurvedic Herbal Hair Growth Serum:

Ingredients:

- 1 tablespoon Jamaican Black Castor Oil

- 1 tablespoon Pumpkin Seed Oil

- 5 drops Rosemary essential oil

- 5 drops Peppermint essential oil

- 5 drops Lavender essential oil

Instructions:

1. In a small glass dropper bottle, combine all the oils and essential oils.

2. Close the bottle tightly and shake well to mix the ingredients thoroughly.

3. To use, apply a few drops of the serum directly to the scalp and massage gently for 2-3 minutes.

4. Leave the serum on overnight or for at least 30 minutes before shampooing as usual.

Ayurveda recipes for Alopecia

1. Ayurvedic Herbal Hair Oil for Alopecia:

Ingredients:

- 1/2 cup coconut oil

- 1/2 cup sesame oil

- 2 tablespoons Bhringraj powder

- 2 tablespoons Brahmi powder

- 1 tablespoon Neem powder

- 1 tablespoon Amla powder

- 5 drops Rosemary essential oil

- 5 drops Lavender essential oil

Instructions:

1. In a saucepan, heat the coconut oil and sesame oil over low heat until warm.

2. Add the Bhringraj, Brahmi, Neem, and Amla powders to the warm oil mixture.

3. Stir the mixture continuously over low heat for 10-15 minutes, allowing the herbs to infuse into the oil.

4. Remove the saucepan from heat and let the oil cool to room temperature.

5. Once cooled, strain the oil using a fine mesh strainer or cheesecloth to remove the herbal residues.

6. Add the Rosemary and Lavender essential oils to the strained herbal oil and mix well.

7. Transfer the infused oil into a clean, dark glass bottle for storage.

8. To use, warm a small amount of the herbal oil in your hands and massage it into the scalp and affected areas of hair loss. Leave it on overnight or for at least 1-2 hours before shampooing as usual.

2. Ayurvedic Herbal Hair Mask for Alopecia:

Ingredients:

- 2 tablespoons Fenugreek powder
- 2 tablespoons Aloe vera gel

- 1 tablespoon Hibiscus powder

- 1 tablespoon Tulsi (Holy Basil) powder

- 1 tablespoon Coconut milk

Instructions:

1. In a small bowl, combine all the ingredients to form a smooth paste.

2. Apply the hair mask evenly to the scalp and affected areas of hair loss.

3. Leave the mask on for 30-60 minutes to allow the herbs to penetrate the scalp and stimulate hair follicles.

4. Rinse the mask out thoroughly with lukewarm water, followed by a gentle shampoo and conditioner.

3. Ayurvedic Herbal Hair Rinse for Alopecia:

Ingredients:

- 2 cups water

- 2 tablespoons Brahmi powder

- 1 tablespoon Shikakai powder

- 1 tablespoon Amla powder

- 1 tablespoon Apple cider vinegar

Instructions:

1. Bring the water to a gentle boil in a small saucepan.

2. Add the Brahmi, Shikakai, and Amla powders to the boiling water.

3. Allow the herbs to steep in the water for 10-15 minutes, then remove the saucepan from the heat.

4. Let the herbal infusion cool to room temperature before straining out the herbs.

5. Add the apple cider vinegar to the herbal infusion and mix well.

6. After shampooing your hair, use the herbal rinse as a final rinse to promote scalp health and stimulate hair growth.

These Ayurvedic recipes and formulations harness the power of natural herbs and botanicals to nourish the scalp, strengthen the hair follicles, and promote healthy hair growth. Incorporating these treatments into your regular hair care routine can help you achieve lustrous, vibrant hair from roots to tips.

Integration into Hair Care Routine:

Incorporating Ayurvedic herbal remedies into our hair care routine requires a thoughtful and consistent approach. By integrating these remedies into our regular practices of oiling, massaging, and cleansing, we can nourish the scalp, strengthen the hair follicles, and promote overall hair health. Consistency is key, as the cumulative effects of these herbal treatments yield long-lasting benefits for hair growth and vitality.

Chapter 4

Ayurvedic Diet and Nutrition for Healthy Hair

The health of our hair is intricately linked to our diet and nutritional intake. In this chapter, we delve into the principles of Ayurvedic diet and nutrition as they pertain to promoting healthy hair growth, preventing hair loss, and maintaining overall hair health.

Understanding the Role of Diet in Hair Health:

Ayurveda recognizes that the foods we consume directly impact the balance of the doshas and the overall functioning of our body, including the health of our hair. A nourishing diet rich in essential nutrients provides the building blocks necessary for strong, lustrous hair, while poor dietary choices can lead to deficiencies and imbalances that manifest as hair-related issues.

Balancing the Doshas:

Ayurvedic dietetics emphasize the importance of balancing the doshas through the consumption of foods that pacify or aggravate each dosha, depending on an individual's unique constitution (Prakriti) and current imbalances (Vikriti). For example:

- Vata-Pacifying Foods: Warm, nourishing foods such as cooked grains, root vegetables, ghee, and warming spices help to ground Vata dosha and prevent dryness and brittleness in the hair.

- Pitta-Pacifying Foods: Cooling, hydrating foods such as leafy greens, cucumbers, coconut, and sweet fruits help to pacify Pitta dosha and reduce inflammation in the scalp, preventing premature graying and hair loss.

- Kapha-Pacifying Foods: Light, dry, and warming foods such as legumes, leafy greens, ginger, and bitter vegetables help to balance Kapha dosha and prevent excessive oiliness and stagnation in the scalp.

Nutrients Essential for Hair Health:

Certain nutrients play a crucial role in supporting healthy hair growth and preventing hair loss. These include:

- Protein: Essential for the formation of keratin, the protein that makes up hair strands. Sources include lean meats, fish, eggs, legumes, and dairy products.

- Omega-3 Fatty Acids: Support scalp health, reduce inflammation, and promote hair growth. Sources include fatty fish, flaxseeds, chia seeds, and walnuts.

- Vitamins and Minerals: Important for hair follicle function and overall hair health. Key vitamins include Vitamin A, C, E, and Biotin, while minerals such as iron, zinc, and selenium are also crucial.

Ayurvedic Dietary Recommendations for Healthy Hair:

- Incorporate a variety of fresh, whole foods into your diet, emphasizing seasonal fruits and vegetables, whole grains, nuts, seeds, and lean proteins.

- Stay hydrated by drinking plenty of water throughout the day, as hydration is essential for maintaining scalp health and promoting hair growth.

- Favor warm, cooked foods over cold or raw foods, as they are easier to digest and assimilate, supporting optimal nutrient absorption.

- Practice mindful eating and avoid overeating, as excessive consumption can lead to digestive imbalances that impact hair health.

Lifestyle Practices for Supporting Hair Health:

In addition to dietary modifications, Ayurveda advocates for lifestyle practices that support overall well-being and promote healthy hair growth. These include:

- Maintaining a regular sleep schedule to ensure adequate rest and rejuvenation for the body and mind.

- Incorporating stress-reducing activities such as yoga, meditation, and deep breathing exercises to manage stress levels, as chronic stress can contribute to hair loss.

- Engaging in regular physical activity to improve circulation, reduce inflammation, and promote overall vitality.

Chapter 5

Lifestyle Practices for Stronger, Healthier Hair

In the pursuit of healthy, vibrant hair, lifestyle factors play a significant role in complementing dietary choices and herbal remedies. In this chapter, we explore the importance of lifestyle practices according to Ayurveda and how they contribute to stronger, healthier hair.

Understanding the Impact of Lifestyle on Hair Health:

Ayurveda recognizes that our lifestyle habits directly influence the balance of the doshas, the strength of our digestive fire (Agni), and the overall functioning of our body, including the health of our hair. By adopting lifestyle practices that support optimal digestion, circulation, and stress management, we can create an environment conducive to healthy hair growth and prevent common hair concerns.

Managing Stress:

Chronic stress is a significant contributing factor to hair loss and other hair-related issues. According to Ayurveda, excess stress disturbs the balance of the doshas, particularly Pitta dosha, leading to inflammation and disruption of hair growth cycles. To manage stress effectively, individuals are encouraged to incorporate stress-reducing activities into their daily routine, such as:

- Yoga: Practicing yoga asanas (poses) and pranayama (breathwork) helps to calm the mind, reduce tension, and promote relaxation.

- Meditation: Daily meditation practice can alleviate stress, improve focus, and enhance overall well-being, supporting healthy hair growth.

- Mindful Awareness: Cultivating mindfulness in daily activities fosters a sense of presence and equanimity, reducing the impact of stress on the body and mind.

Balancing Work and Rest:

Balancing periods of activity with adequate rest and relaxation is essential for maintaining overall health and vitality, including hair health. Ayurveda emphasizes the importance of establishing a regular daily routine (Dinacharya) that includes:

- Adequate Sleep: Aim for 7-9 hours of quality sleep each night to allow the body to rest, repair, and rejuvenate. Establishing a consistent sleep schedule promotes optimal functioning of the body's natural rhythms, including hair growth cycles.

- Work-Life Balance: Strive to maintain a healthy balance between work, leisure, and self-care activities. Prioritize time for relaxation, hobbies, and activities that bring joy and fulfillment, reducing stress and promoting overall well-being.

Supporting Digestive Health:

Optimal digestion is essential for the absorption and assimilation of nutrients necessary for healthy hair growth. Ayurveda recommends adopting lifestyle practices that support robust digestion, including:

- Eating Mindfully: Practice mindful eating by savoring each bite, chewing food thoroughly, and avoiding distractions during meals. This enhances digestion and promotes nutrient absorption.

- Regular Meal Times: Establish regular meal times and avoid skipping meals, as irregular eating patterns can disrupt digestive function and impact nutrient assimilation.

- Digestive Fire (Agni): Support the strength of digestive fire by consuming warming spices such as ginger, cumin, and black pepper, and by avoiding heavy, processed foods that burden digestion.

Promoting Scalp Health:

Maintaining a healthy scalp environment is crucial for optimal hair growth and preventing scalp-related issues such as dandruff and inflammation. Ayurvedic lifestyle practices that support scalp health include:

- Scalp Massage: Regular scalp massage with warm herbal oils stimulates circulation, nourishes the hair follicles, and promotes relaxation. Use gentle circular motions to distribute oil evenly and enhance absorption.

- Herbal Hair Care: Incorporate Ayurvedic herbal shampoos, conditioners, and hair masks into your hair care routine to cleanse, nourish, and rejuvenate the scalp and hair follicles.

Chapter 6

Ayurvedic Hair Care Routines: Nurturing Your Scalp and Hair

A consistent and mindful hair care routine is essential for maintaining scalp health, promoting hair growth, and preserving the natural beauty of your hair. In this chapter, we explore Ayurvedic hair care practices and rituals that nourish the scalp, strengthen the hair follicles, and enhance overall hair health.

Understanding the Importance of Scalp Health:

In Ayurveda, the scalp is considered the foundation of healthy hair growth. A balanced and nourished scalp creates an optimal environment for hair follicles to thrive, while imbalances or disturbances in the scalp can lead to various hair concerns such as dandruff, dryness, and hair loss. By prioritizing scalp health in your hair care routine, you can support the growth of strong, lustrous hair from the roots.

Ayurvedic Hair Care Rituals:

1. Scalp Massage (Abhyanga): Regular scalp massage with warm herbal oils is a cornerstone of Ayurvedic hair care. This practice stimulates circulation, enhances nutrient delivery to the hair follicles, and promotes relaxation. Use gentle circular motions to massage the scalp for 5-10 minutes before bedtime or prior to showering.

2. Oil Treatment (Shiro Abhyanga): Applying herbal hair oils to the scalp and hair is a nourishing ritual that strengthens the roots, conditions the hair shaft, and prevents dryness and breakage. Choose oils based on your hair type and needs, such as Bhringraj oil for promoting hair growth or Brahmi oil for calming the scalp.

3. Herbal Hair Wash (Shampooing): Choose Ayurvedic herbal shampoos and cleansers that are gentle on the scalp and free from harsh chemicals. Look for ingredients such as Shikakai, Amla, and Neem, which cleanse the scalp, remove impurities, and promote healthy hair growth.

4. Conditioning Treatments: Incorporate natural conditioning treatments such as herbal hair masks, yogurt, or aloe vera gel to hydrate the hair, improve manageability, and add shine. Customize your conditioning treatments based on your hair's needs, such as using Amla powder for strengthening or Hibiscus for adding volume.

5. Detoxification (Scalp Scrubs): Periodically exfoliate the scalp with gentle scalp scrubs or herbal pastes to remove dead skin cells, excess oil, and product buildup. This helps to unclog hair follicles, promote circulation, and maintain a healthy scalp environment.

Tailoring Your Hair Care Routine:

- Identify Your Hair Type: Determine your hair type (Vata, Pitta, or Kapha predominant) and choose hair care products and practices that align with your unique needs and imbalances.

- Consider Seasonal Adjustments: Adapt your hair care routine to the changing seasons, as environmental factors such as temperature, humidity, and sunlight can impact scalp health and hair growth.

- Listen to Your Hair: Pay attention to how your hair responds to different products and treatments, and adjust your routine accordingly. Trust your intuition and prioritize practices that leave your hair feeling nourished, balanced, and vibrant.

Chapter 7

Ayurvedic Remedies for Common Hair Concerns

1. Dandruff and Scalp Irritation:

- Neem and Tea Tree Oil Scalp Treatment: Neem and tea tree oil have potent antimicrobial properties that help combat fungal infections and soothe scalp irritation. Mix neem oil with a few drops of tea tree oil and massage into the scalp. Leave on for 30 minutes before shampooing.

2. Hair Loss and Thinning:

- Bhringraj Hair Oil: Bhringraj oil is renowned for its hair-strengthening properties and is particularly effective in combating hair loss and promoting regrowth. Massage warm Bhringraj oil into the scalp and leave it on overnight for best results.

3. Premature Graying:

- Amla and Curry Leaf Hair Mask: Amla is rich in antioxidants and vitamin C, while curry leaves contain compounds that help restore pigment to the hair. Make a paste with Amla powder, curry leaves, and water. Apply to the hair and scalp, leave on for 30 minutes, then rinse.

4. Lack of Volume and Luster:

- Hibiscus and Fenugreek Hair Rinse: Hibiscus strengthens hair follicles and adds shine, while fenugreek boosts volume and texture. Steep dried hibiscus flowers and fenugreek seeds in hot water for 30 minutes. Strain, cool, and use as a final hair rinse after shampooing.

5. Oily Scalp and Greasy Hair:

- Shikakai and Lemon Scalp Cleanser: Shikakai acts as a natural cleanser, while lemon helps balance oil production on the scalp. Mix shikakai powder with fresh lemon juice to form a paste. Apply to the scalp and hair, leave on for 15 minutes, then rinse thoroughly.

6. Dry and Damaged Hair:

- Coconut Milk and Aloe Vera Hair Mask: Coconut milk moisturizes and nourishes the hair, while aloe vera soothes and repairs damage. Blend fresh coconut milk with aloe vera gel and apply to the hair and scalp. Leave on for 30 minutes, then shampoo as usual.

7. Split Ends and Breakage:

- Castor Oil and Rosemary Serum: Castor oil strengthens hair strands and reduces breakage, while rosemary stimulates circulation to the scalp. Mix castor oil with a few drops of rosemary essential oil and apply to the ends of the hair. Leave on overnight for intensive treatment.

8. Lack of Hair Growth:

- Fenugreek and Onion Juice Scalp Treatment: Fenugreek seeds are rich in protein and nutrients that promote hair growth, while onion juice contains sulfur, which helps nourish hair follicles. Soak fenugreek seeds overnight, blend with fresh onion juice, and apply to the scalp. Leave on for 30 minutes before shampooing.

- Rosemary and Clove Hair Oil: Rosemary stimulates blood circulation to the scalp, promoting hair growth and strengthening hair follicles. Cloves have antimicrobial properties that help maintain scalp health and prevent dandruff and other scalp infections. Add dry rosemary leaves and whole cloves to warm carrier oil(coconut oil or jojoba oil). Let the herbs infuse into the oil for 30 minutes. Strain and apply infused oil to your scalp and massage gently. Leave oil on for at least 30minutes or overnight for maximum benefit . Wash you hair with shampoo and conditioner as usual.

9. Itchy Scalp:

- Mint and Aloe Vera Scalp Soothing Mask: Mint has cooling properties that alleviate itchiness and inflammation, while aloe vera hydrates and calms the scalp. Mix crushed mint leaves with fresh aloe vera gel and apply to the scalp. Leave on for 20 minutes before rinsing.

10. Lack of Shine and Gloss:

- Yogurt and Honey Hair Mask: Yogurt contains lactic acid, which helps cleanse and exfoliate the scalp, while honey locks in moisture and adds shine. Mix plain yogurt with honey and apply to the hair and scalp. Leave on for 30 minutes before rinsing with lukewarm water.

11. Environmental Damage Protection:

- Coconut Oil and Vitamin E Hair Serum: Coconut oil provides a protective barrier against environmental damage, while vitamin E nourishes and strengthens hair. Mix coconut oil with vitamin E oil and apply sparingly to the hair, focusing on the ends. Leave on overnight for intensive repair.

12. Sun Damage Repair:

- Aloe Vera and Coconut Milk Hair Mask: Aloe vera soothes sun-damaged scalp and hair, while coconut milk hydrates and repairs UV damage. Blend fresh aloe vera gel with coconut milk and apply to the hair and scalp. Leave on for 1 hour before rinsing with cool water.

13. Chemical Damage Recovery:

- Avocado and Banana Hair Mask: Avocado provides essential fatty acids that nourish and repair damaged hair, while banana restores elasticity and softness. Mash ripe avocado and banana together and apply to the hair. Leave on for 30 minutes before rinsing thoroughly.

14. Environmental Pollution Protection:

- Green Tea and Apple Cider Vinegar Rinse: Green tea contains antioxidants that protect against environmental pollutants, while apple cider vinegar balances pH and clarifies the scalp. Steep green tea in hot water, cool, and mix with apple cider vinegar. Use as a final rinse after shampooing.

15. Stress-Induced Hair Loss:

- Chamomile and Lavender Scalp Massage Oil: Chamomile and

lavender have calming properties that help reduce stress and promote relaxation, supporting healthy hair growth. Infuse chamomile and lavender flowers in warm coconut oil and massage into the scalp. Leave on overnight for maximum benefit.

By incorporating these additional Ayurvedic remedies into your hair care routine, you can address a wide range of hair concerns and maintain vibrant, healthy hair naturally. Each remedy is tailored to target specific issues, providing holistic support for your scalp and hair health.

www.ingramcontent.com/pod-product-compliance
Lightning Source LLC
Chambersburg PA
CBHW051855250726
48659CB00006B/2215